#VET RECEPTIONIST LIFE

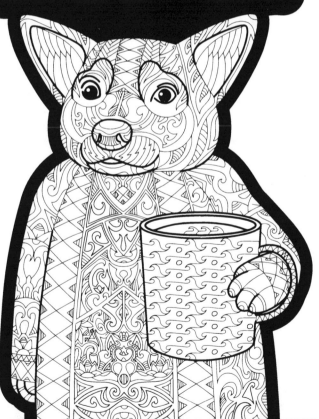

VET RECEPTIONIST COLORING BOOK WITH ANIMAL MANDALAS

Thank you for choosing us!

We hope you enjoy this purchase :)

As a small business selling only on Amazon, your feedback is the

upmost importance to us.

If you could take a minute to post a review on Amazon,

we would so appreciate it!

Love M.P x

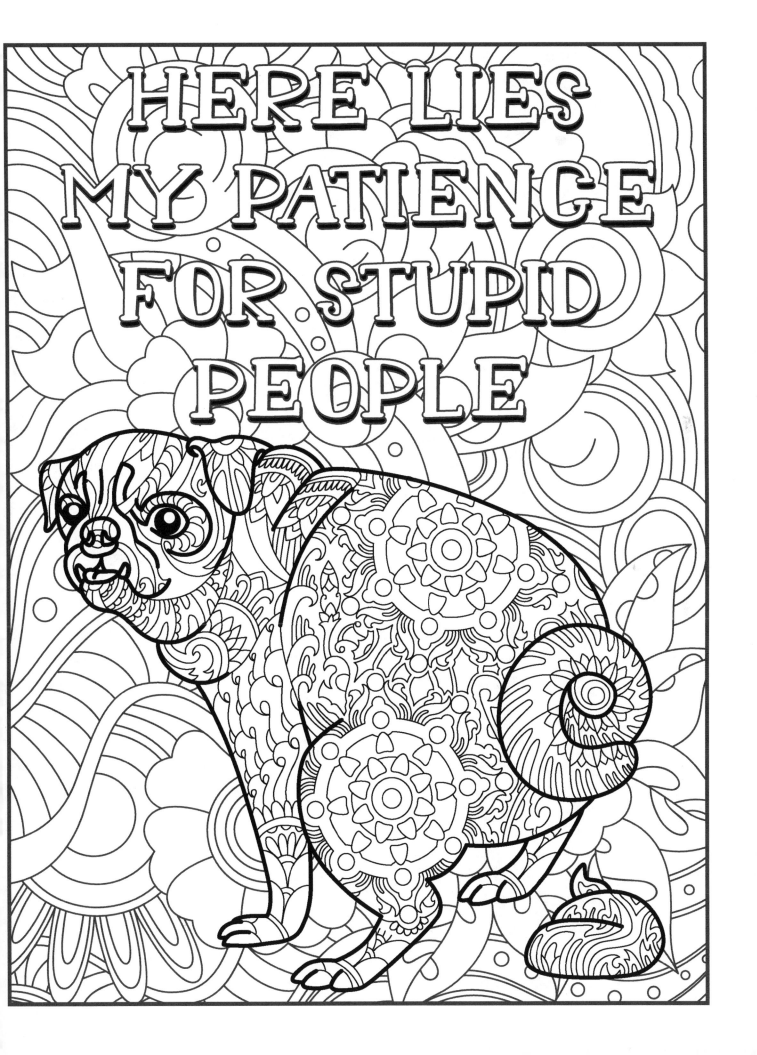

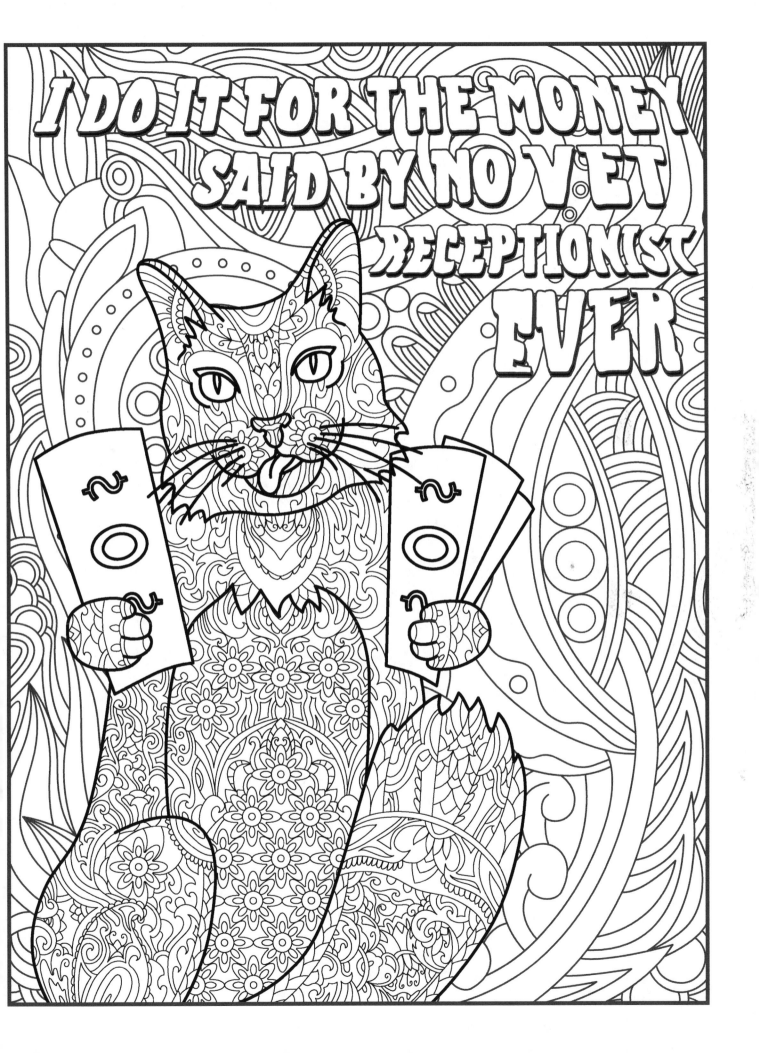

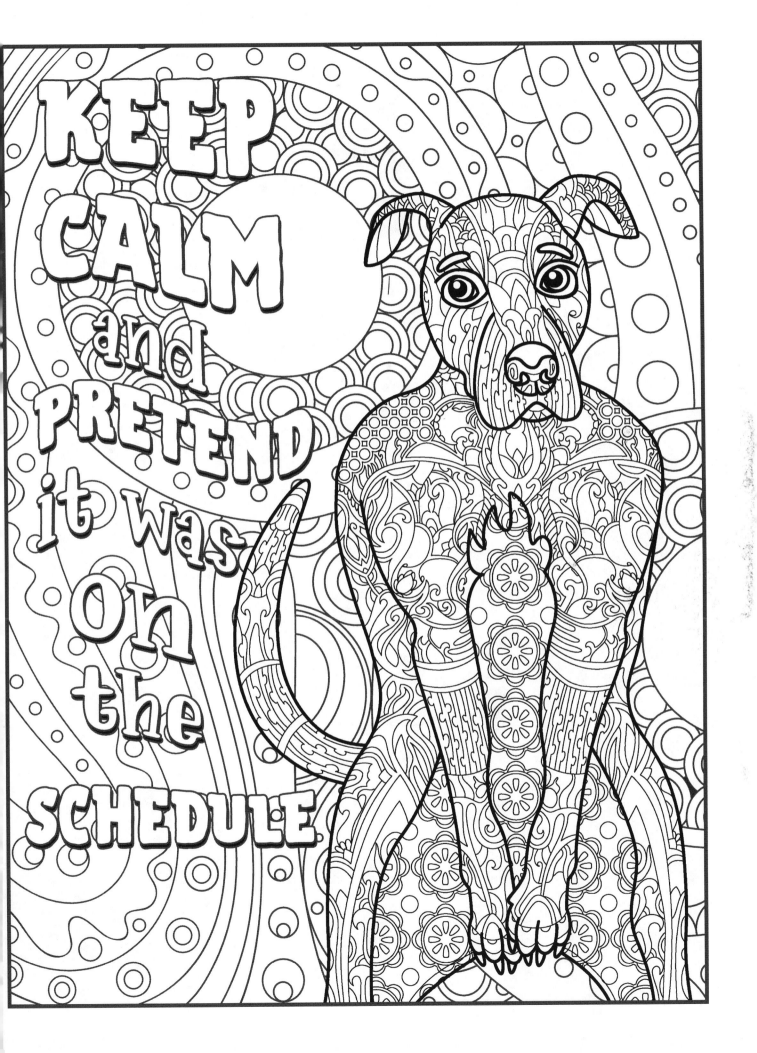

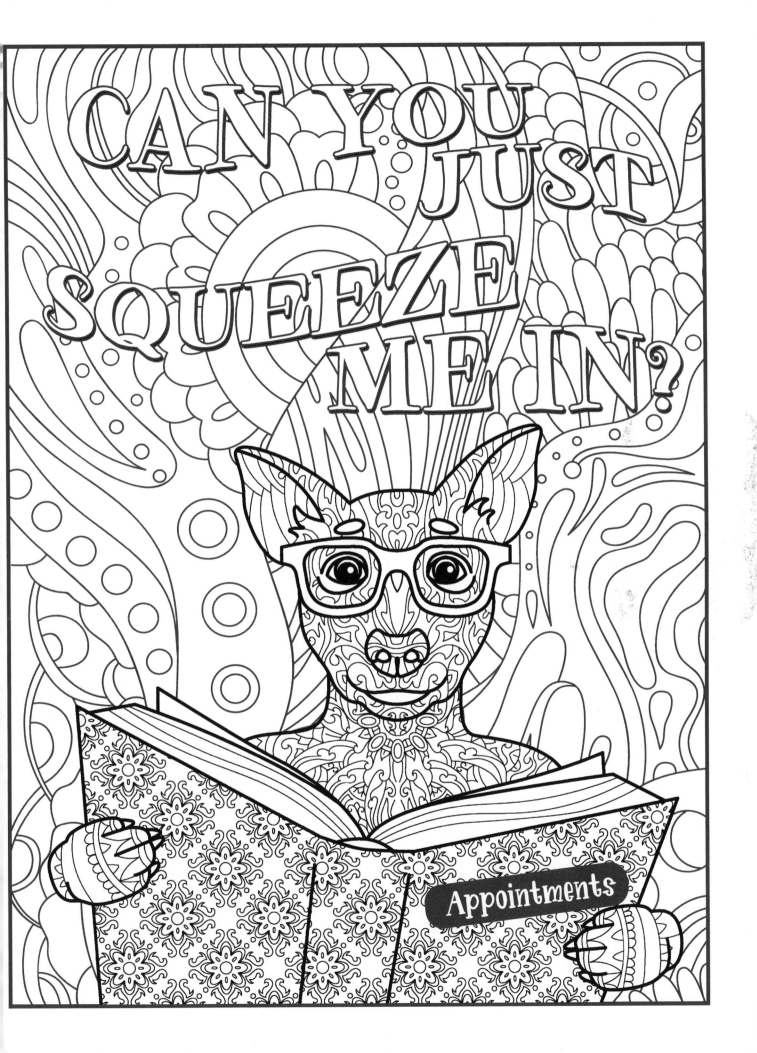

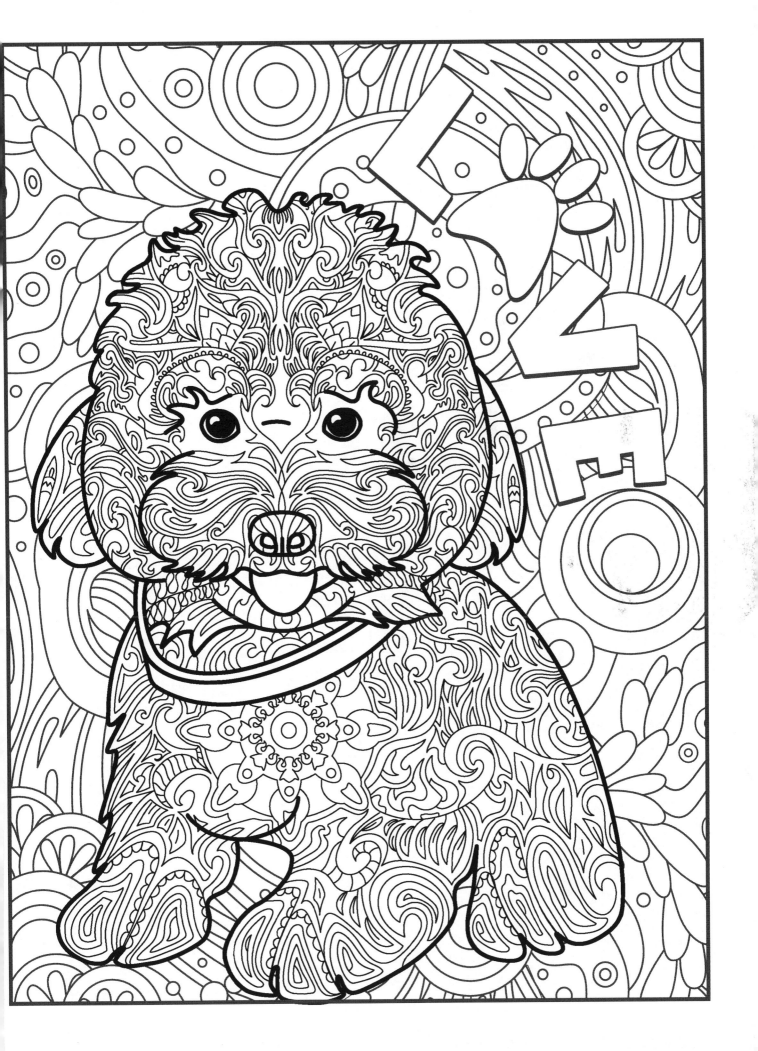

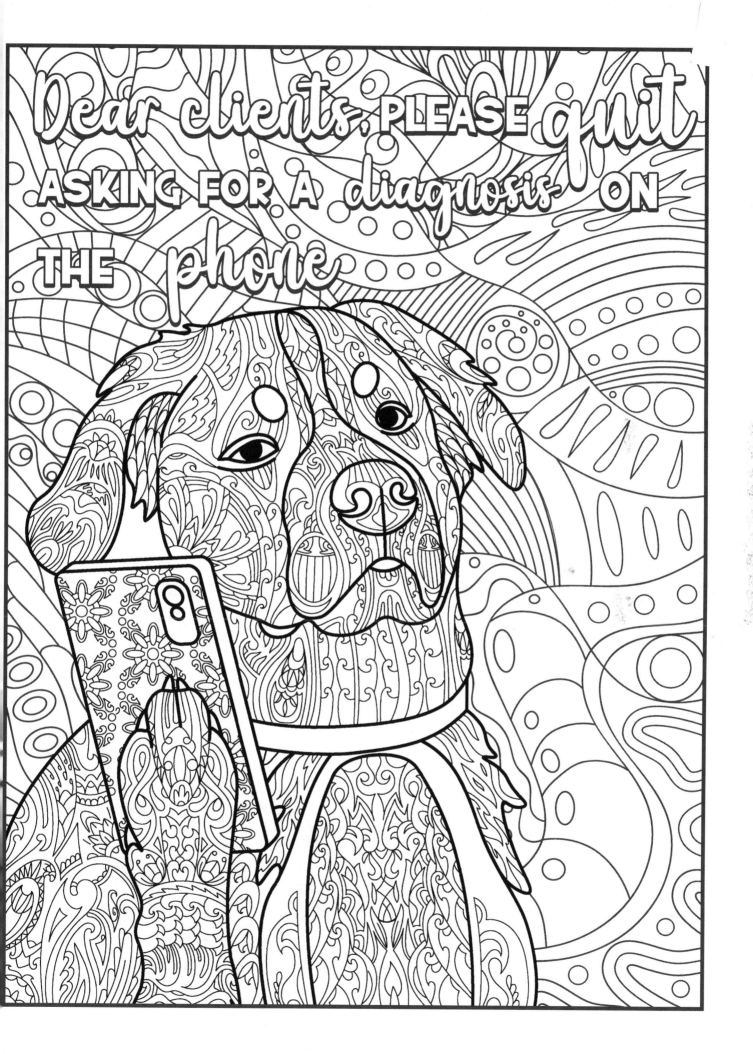

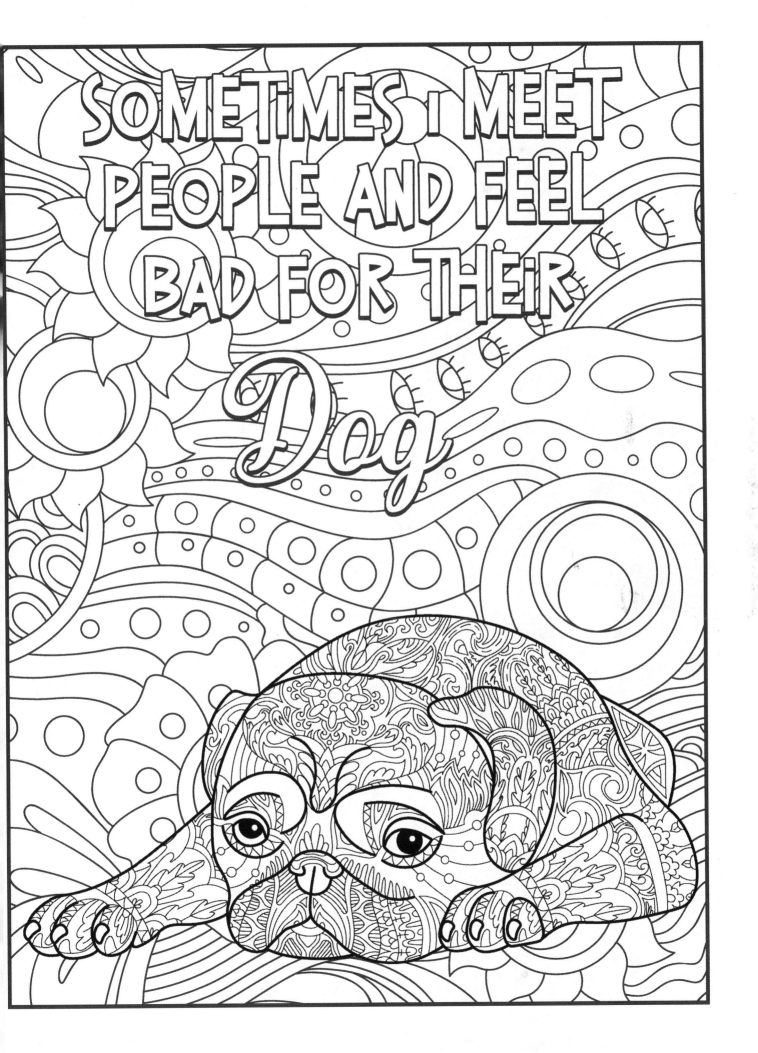

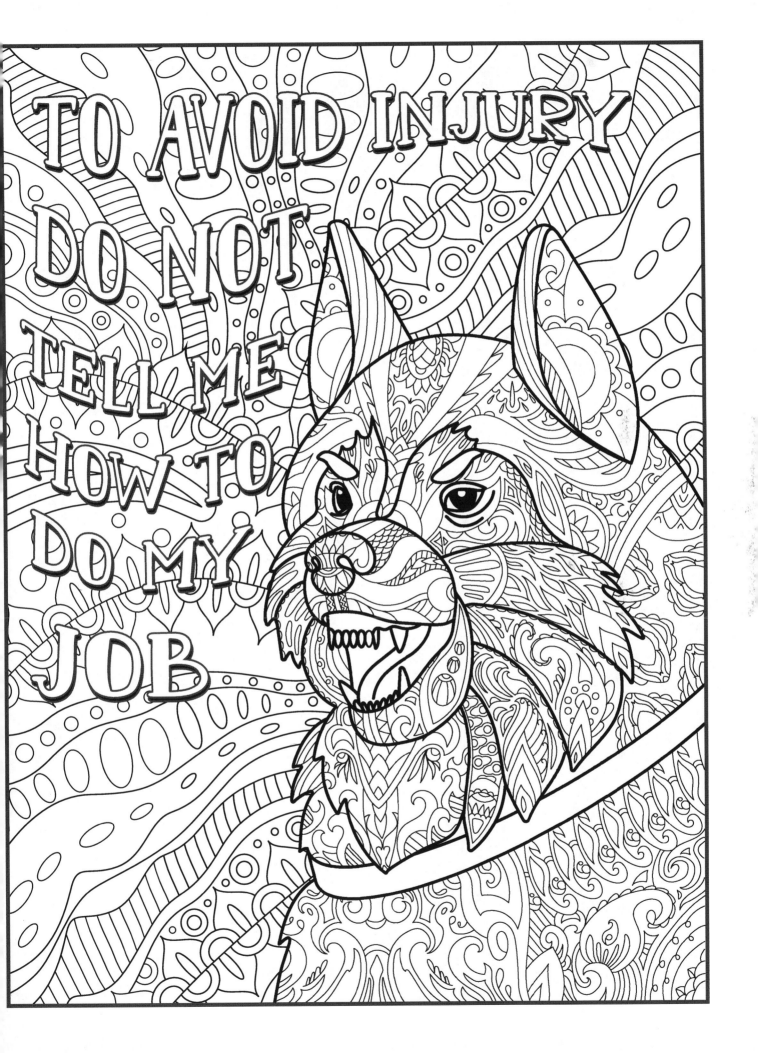

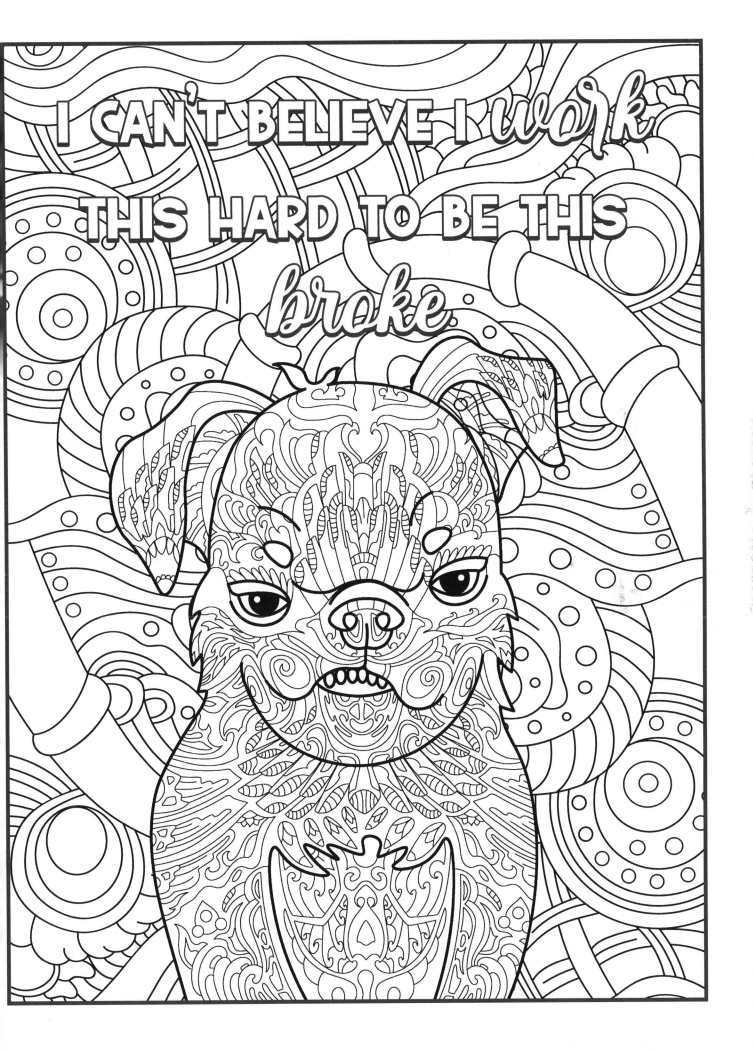

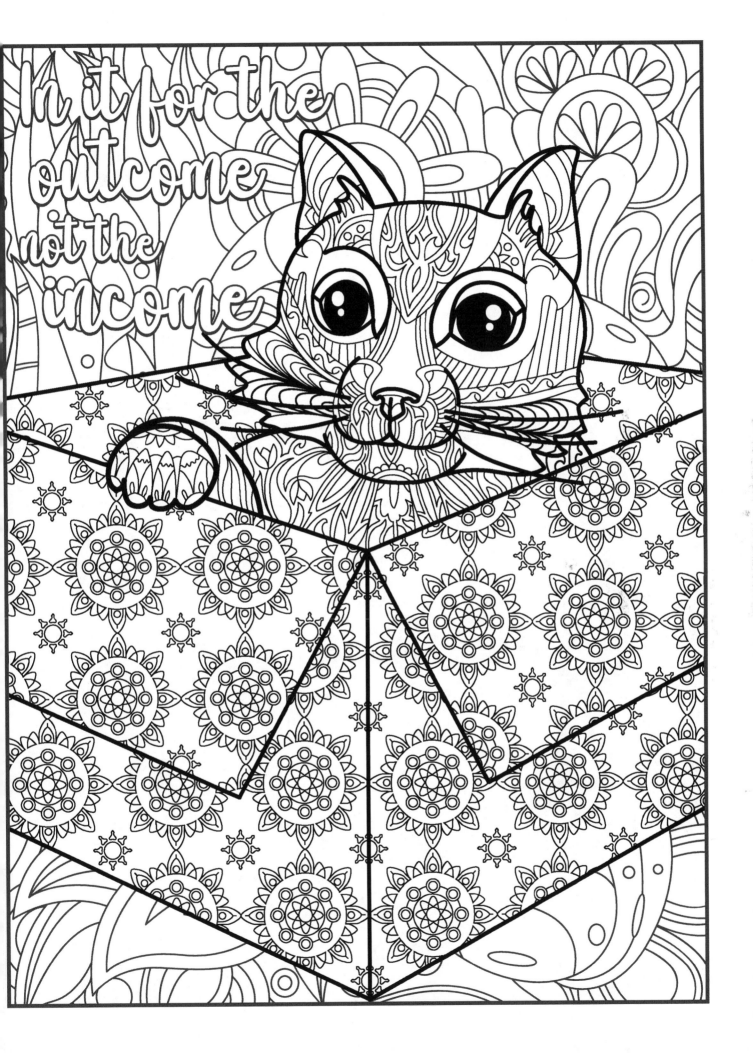

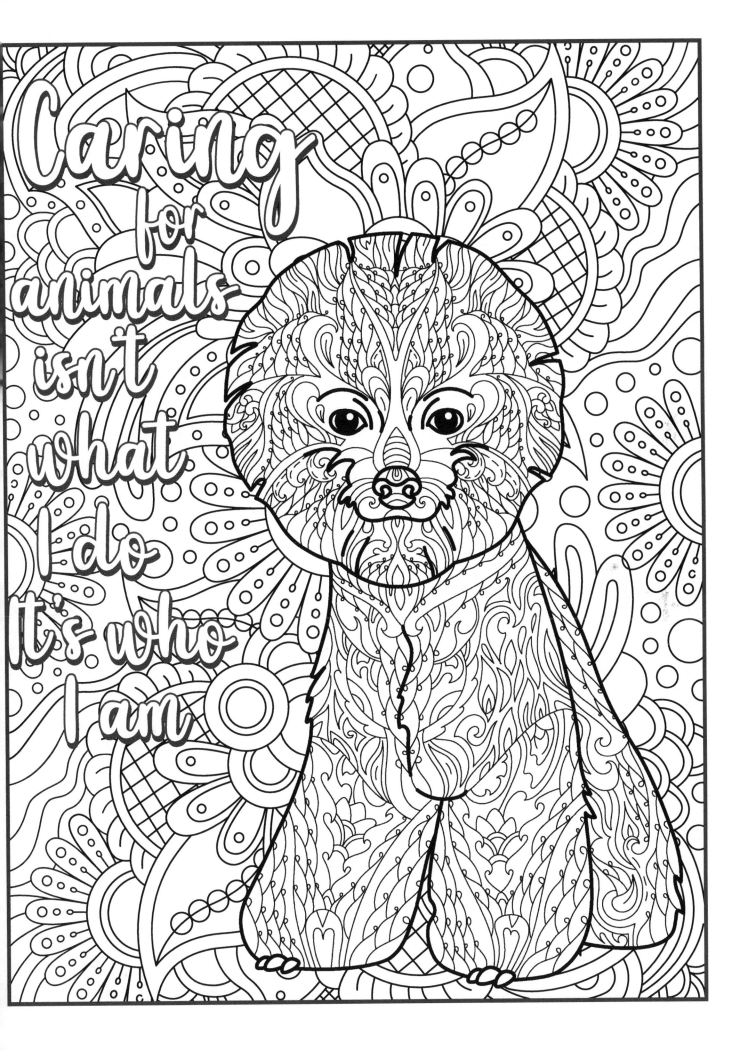

Caring for animals isn't what I do It's who I am

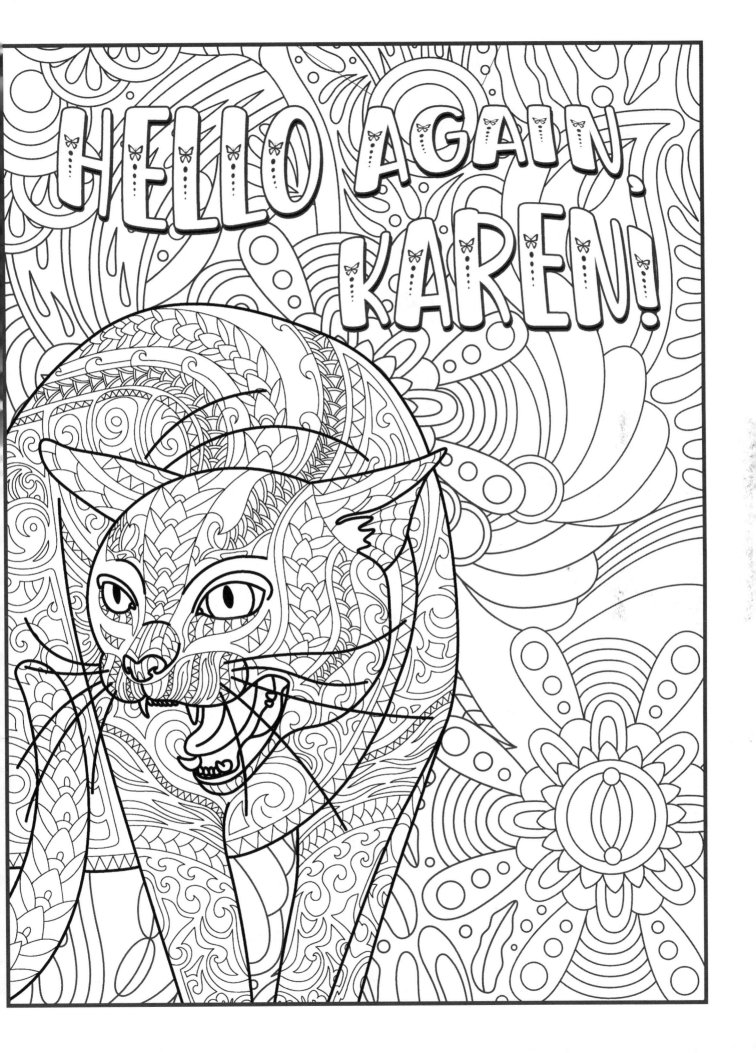

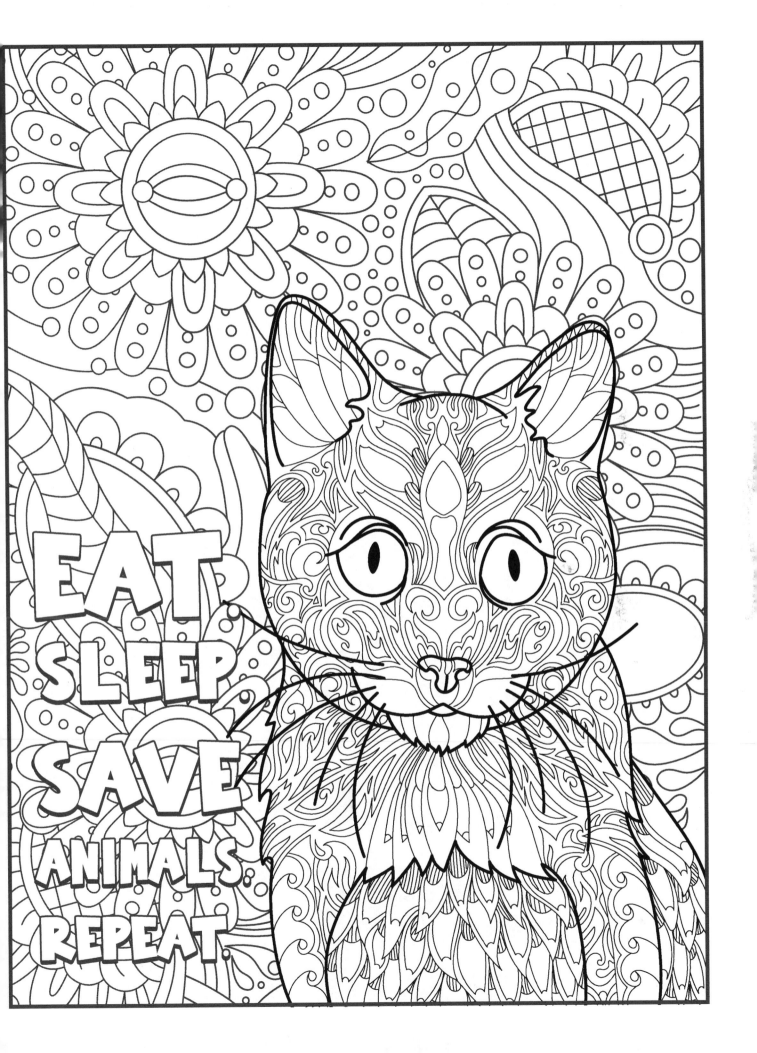

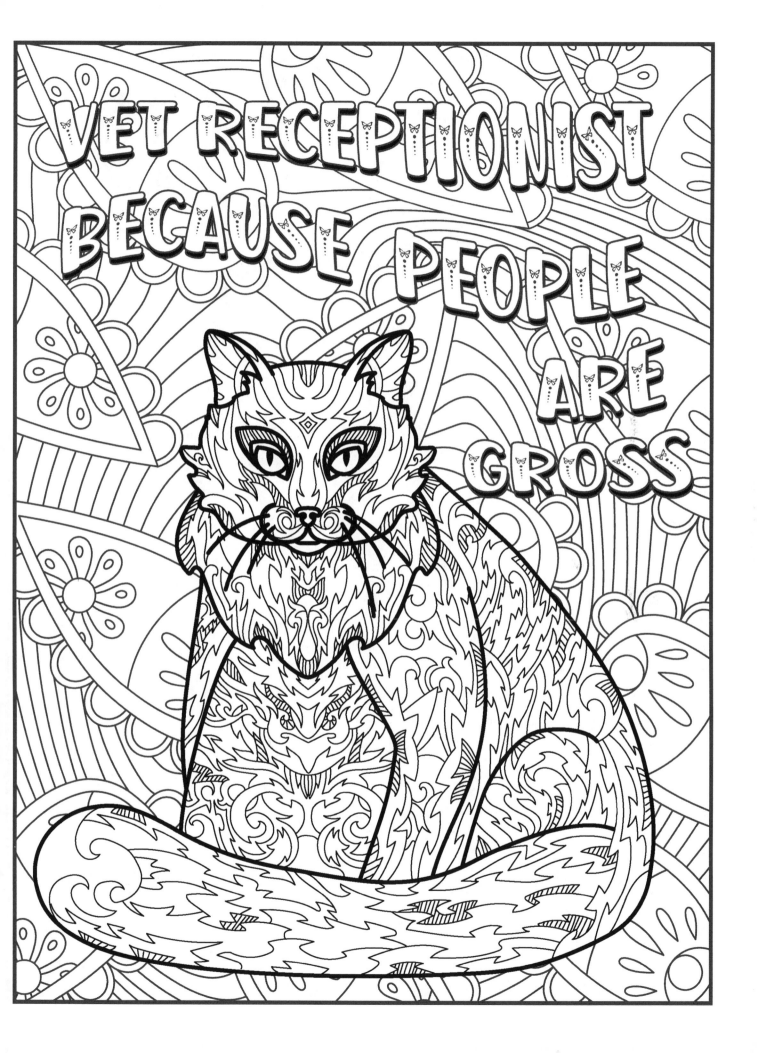

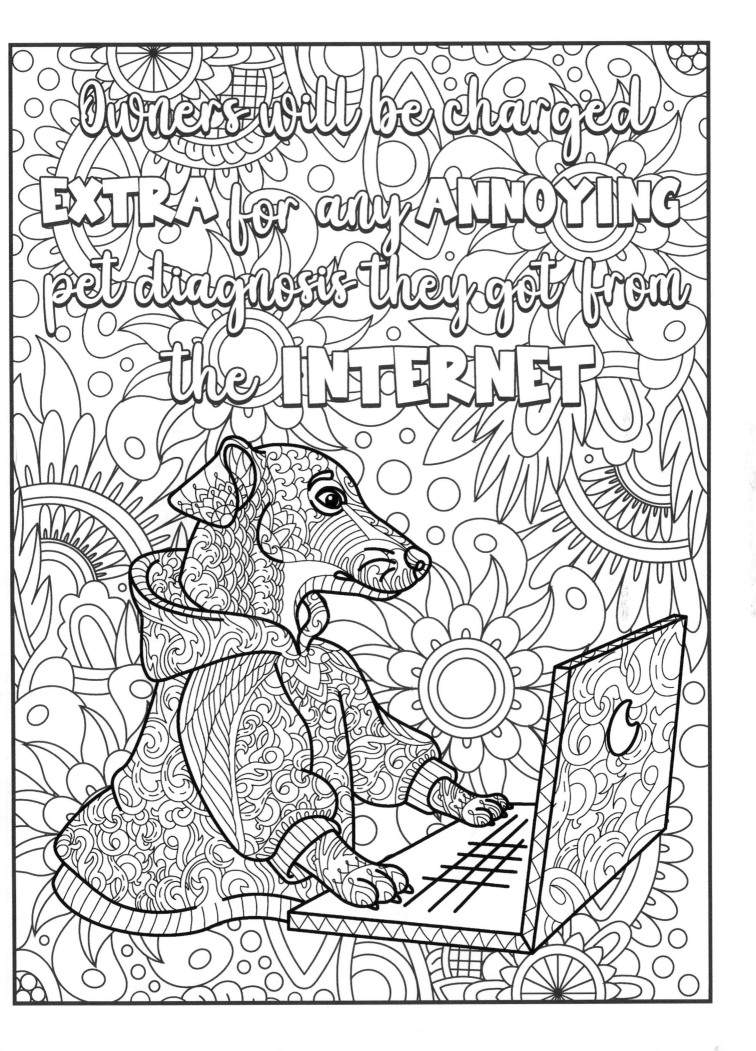

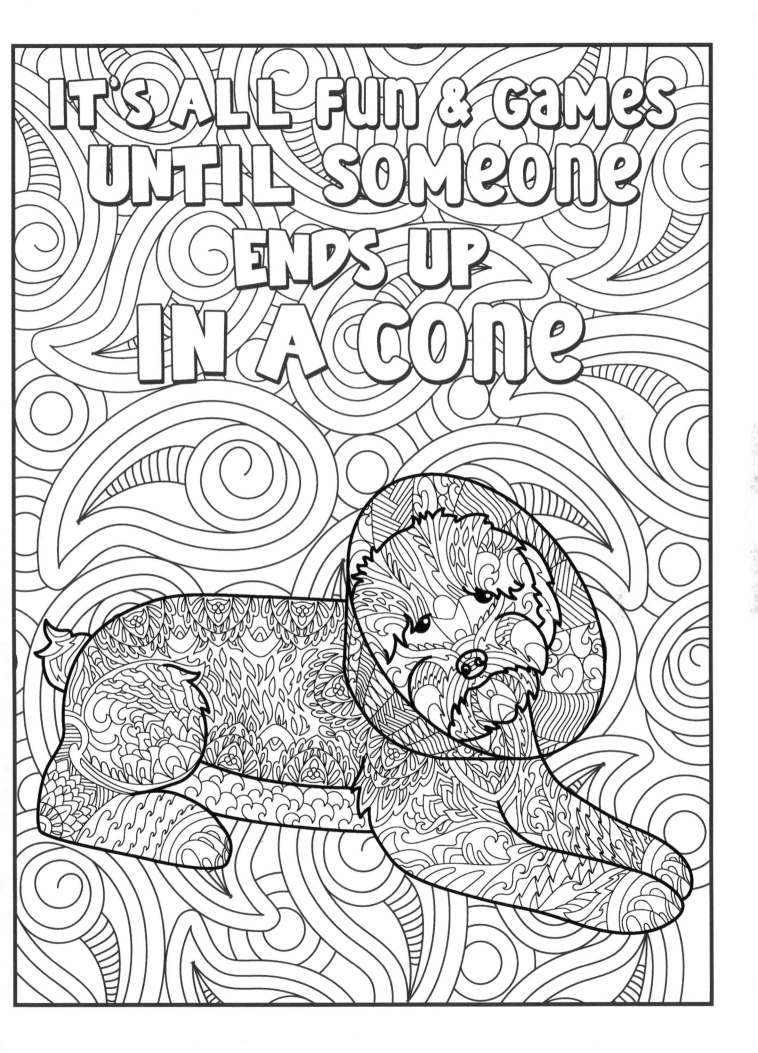

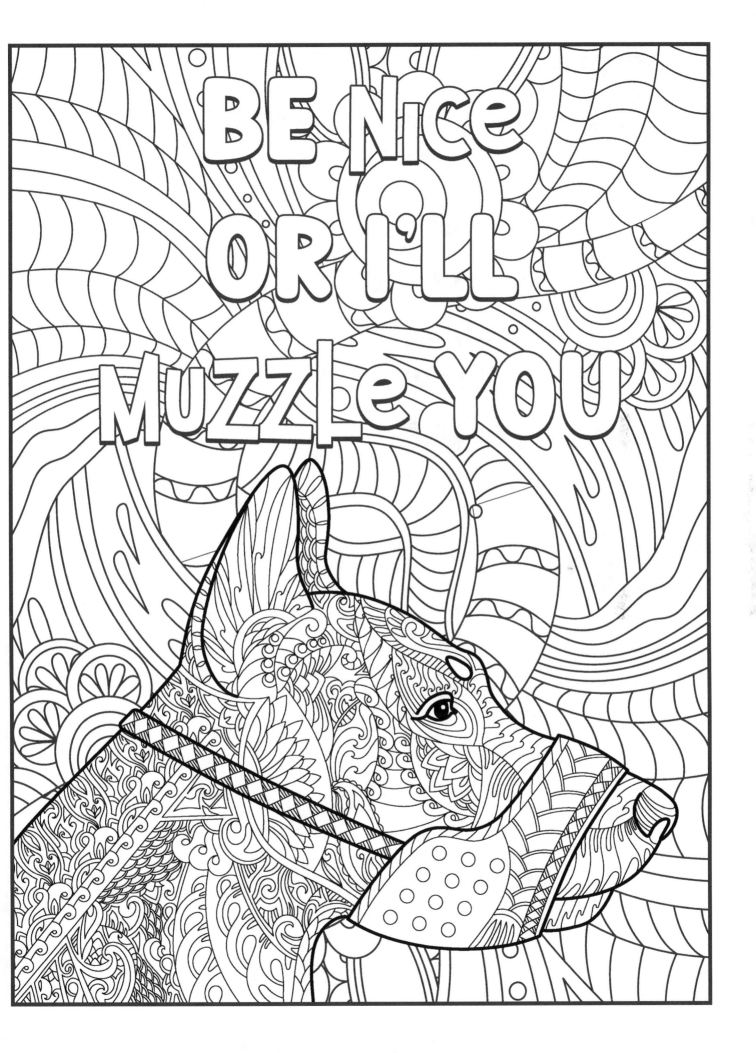

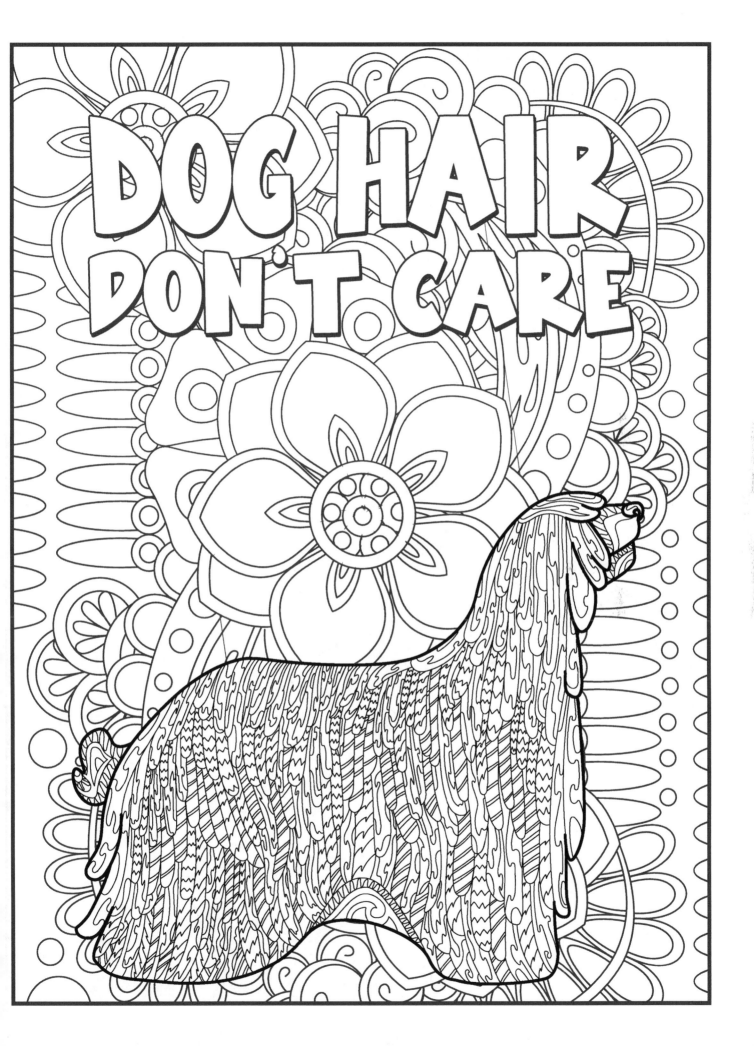

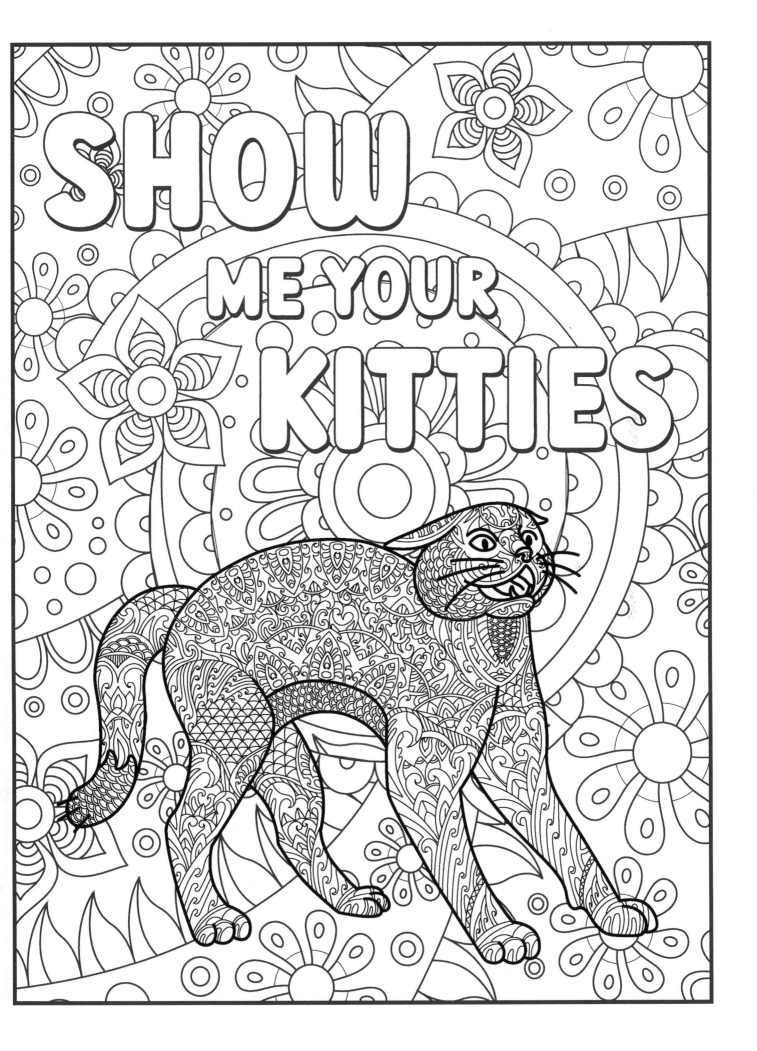

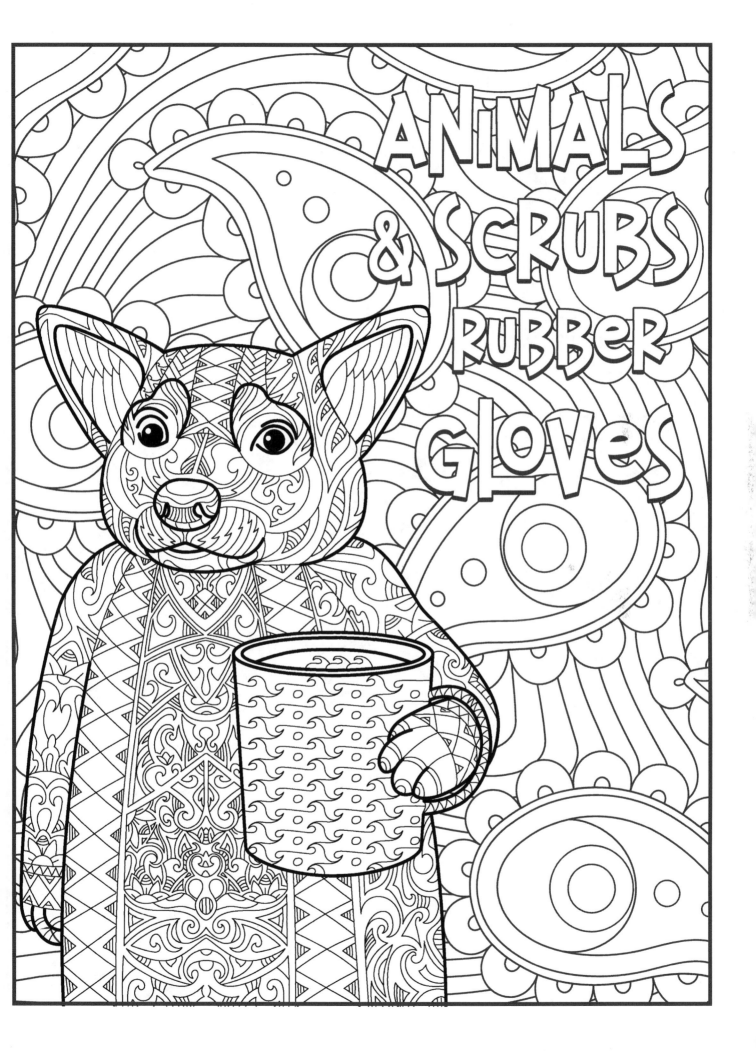

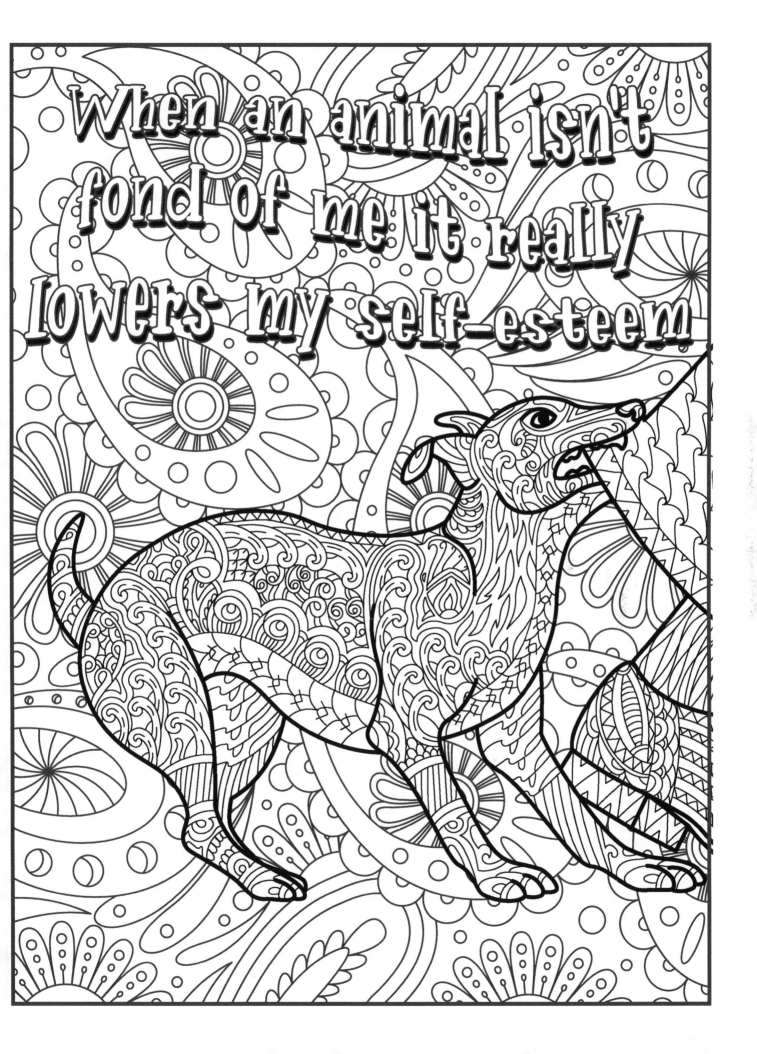

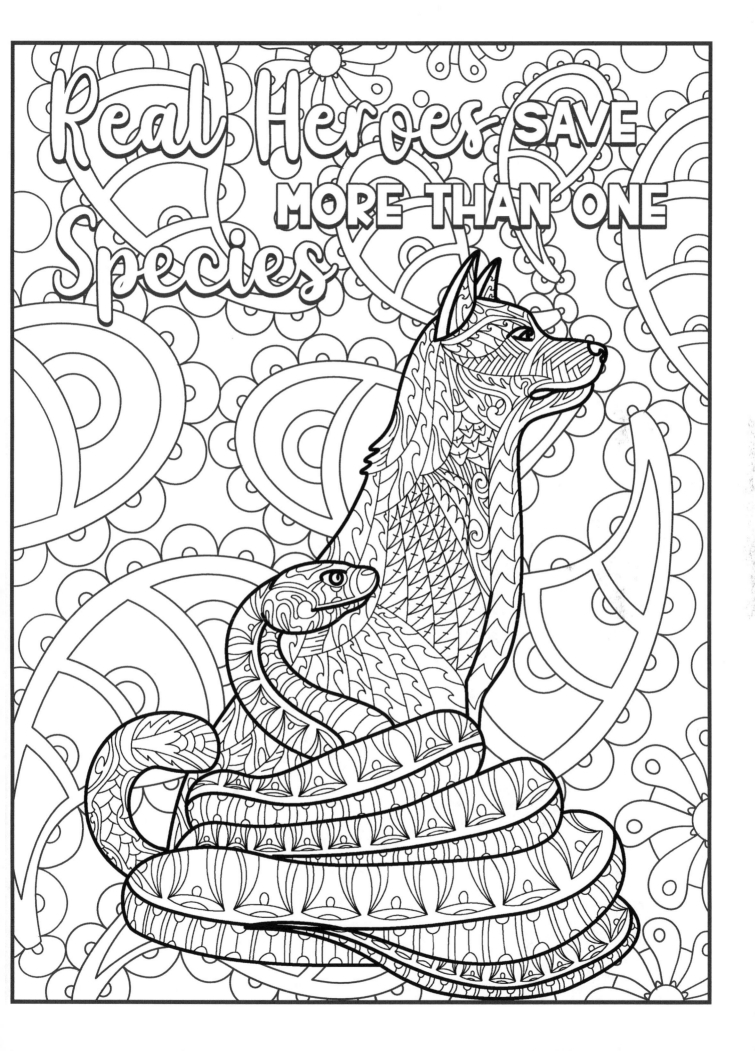

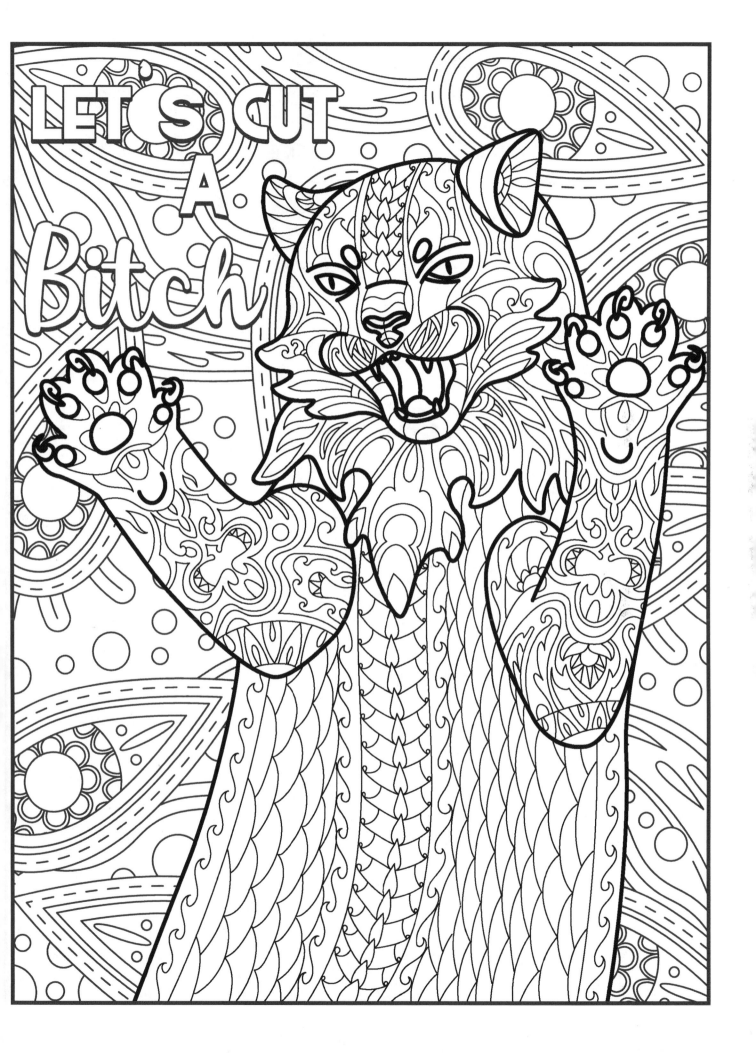

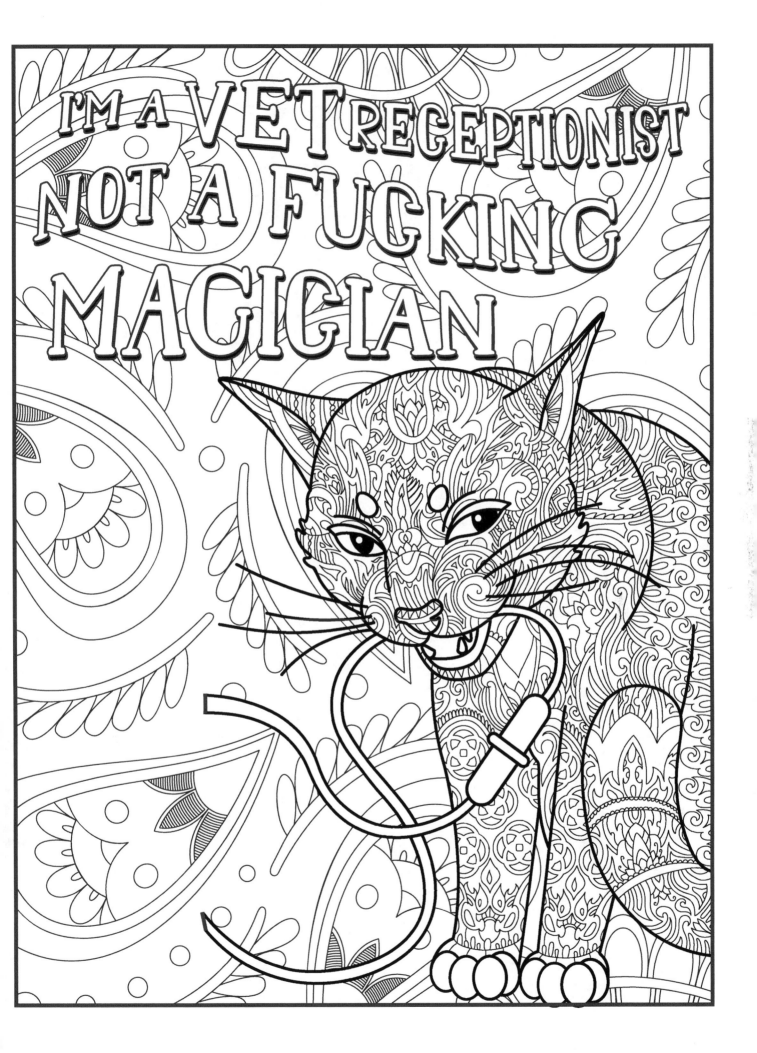

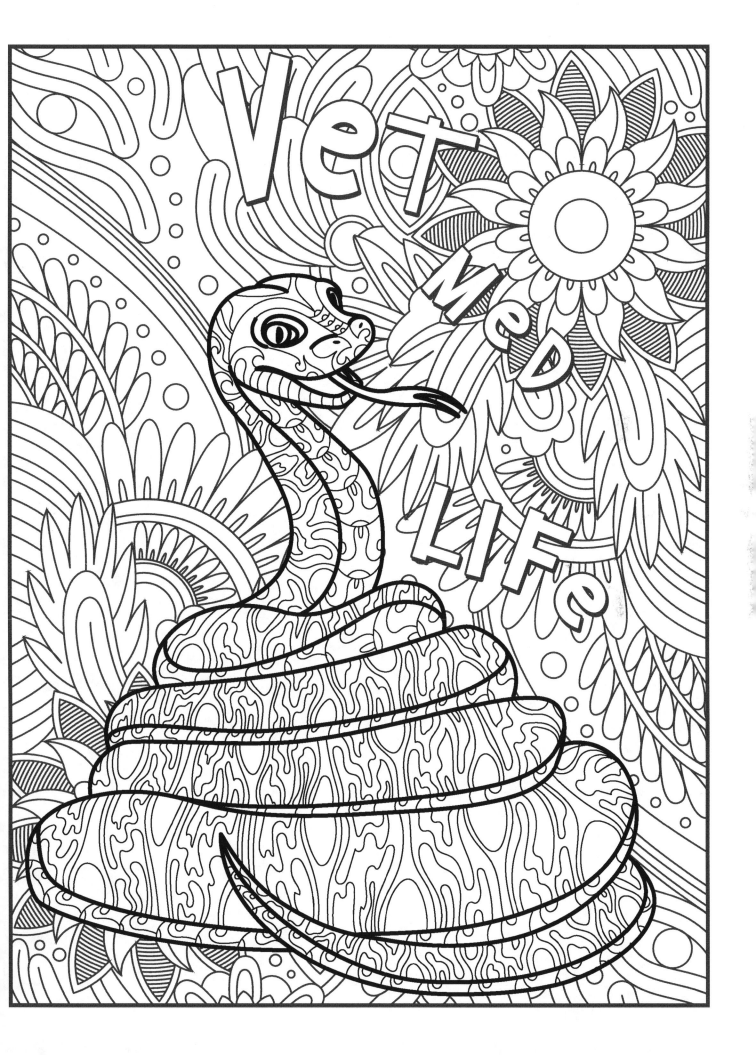

Thank you for choosing us!

We hope you enjoy this purchase :)

As a small business selling only on Amazon, your feedback is the

upmost importance to us.

If you could take a minute to post a review on Amazon,

we would so appreciate it!

Love M.P x

Made in the USA
Columbia, SC
19 October 2023

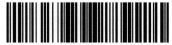

24693068R00030